Getting Past the Fear

A guide to help you mentally prepare for chemotherapy

Nancy Stordahl

Getting Past the Fear: A guide to help you mentally prepare for chemotherapy, first edition. All rights reserved.

Copyright © 2014 by Nancy Stordahl

Printed in the United States of America

The material presented in this book is not intended to be a substitute for professional medical advice.

ISBN - 10: 0615955924

ISBN - 13: 978-0615955926

Testimonials

"Nancy Stordahl continues with her excellent service to cancer patients and their loved ones in her book, *Getting Past the Fear.* Simply written and always accessible, it provides a much-needed service for both patients and caregivers who will be heading into the chemo experience for the first time. Nancy demystifies what can often seem so daunting and her direct approach is both honest and supportive."

- David Tabatsky, author, *Write for Life: Communicating Your Way Through Cancer* and co-author, *Chicken Soup for the Soul's The Cancer Book: 101 Stories of Courage, Support & Love*

"Getting Past the Fear helped me tremendously. Before chemo I was terrified in a way I had not ever experienced - like an animal. *Getting Past the Fear* helped me put a more rational fence around the chemo experience. I poured over the positive suggestions and followed many of them. Looking back, I realize how helpful this book was. Thanks, Nancy."

- Donna, cancer survivor

"Getting Past the Fear is a wealth of useful information for cancer patients and their families."

- Niki Barr, PhD, author of *Emotional Wellness: The Other Half of Treating Cancer*

"This excellent must-read will be a tremendous help to those about to undergo or undergoing chemotherapy."

- Beth Gainer, cancer survivor and author of the blog, *Calling the Shots.*

For my mother and also for my friend, Rachel. We will not forget.

CONTENTS

Thank you to my family for helping me face the fear, the chemo and all the rest. Special thanks to Lindsay for encouraging me to write this book and to Peter and Aaron for never flinching in their support. Above all, thank you to David for his unwavering love and support in all things.

INTRODUCTION

Have you heard the words, *you have cancer?*

Have you also heard the words, *you need chemotherapy?*

Are you feeling stunned, overwhelmed and afraid?

You are not alone.

Many others have been there. I've been there too. I've felt the fear. If you are facing chemo for the first time, I want to help you get past your fear - at least a little bit past it.

Because sometimes even a little turns out to be a lot.

Nothing is so much to be feared as fear.

Henry David Thoreau, 1851

1

SO YOU NEED CHEMO

When you hear the words, *you have cancer*, life as you knew it is over. It just is. There is no going back. I often compare it to the divide between childhood and adulthood. When you leave childhood behind, you are finished with it forever. You can't go back, only your memories remain. That very special and almost magical childhood innocence is gone for good.

It's the same with cancer. Once you've been diagnosed, another kind of innocence is lost. The healthy body you once knew and probably took for granted suddenly feels fragile and a whole lot more unreliable. You might even feel as if your body has betrayed you, especially if you have always considered yourself to be physically fit and strong. A cancer diagnosis shakes you up not only physically, but emotionally as well. Suddenly everything is changed. Suddenly uncertainty abounds.

Following my breast cancer diagnosis in 2010, there were a few more bombshells yet to come. I tested positive for the BRCA2 gene mutation. I faced the reality of a bilateral mastectomy, or as some refer to it, breast amputations. My bilateral mastectomy was followed by a slow and sometimes painful reconstruction process. Later I faced a total hysterectomy and bilateral salpingo oophorectomy. These things were far from a walk in the park, but nothing quite rattled me more than the realization I would need chemotherapy. The day after my bilateral when my surgeon walked into the room and casually announced that more than likely I would be needing chemotherapy, was almost worse than the day I learned I had cancer. Almost.

Chemotherapy epitomizes cancer at its very worst. Chemotherapy represents everyone's worst cancer nightmare, well, other than the dying part of course. Why is this?

Chemotherapy screams illness. Chemotherapy doesn't let you pretend anymore. Chemotherapy forces you to confront your illness like nothing else does. Chemotherapy forces you to admit you have a serious illness and makes it obvious to the rest of the world (though this is not always the case – and this creates another completely different set of difficult circumstances) as well. There can be no more hiding. Your self-confidence, self-image and general ability to cope are called into question. Chemotherapy literally and figuratively strips you down to your bare essence. Is this an exaggeration? I don't think it is.

In short, chemotherapy makes you vulnerable and this is perhaps why it is so frightening. No one likes to feel afraid and vulnerable; no wonder chemo is so dreaded. In addition, there are the horror stories many of us carry with us in our minds. Many of us have known others who have suffered through the rigors of chemo treatment. Many of us have known others grappling with extreme side effects like nausea, fatigue and hair loss to name a few. Thankfully, many side effects are far more manageable today, but this doesn't mean we don't remember or imagine the worst and sadly, some do still experience the worst possible side effects.

Even if one receives a chemo drug that does not produce the more obvious outward side effects such as hair loss, the reality of needing chemo is a tough pill to swallow. Pun intended.

I don't say these things to minimize other treatments. I would never wish to marginalize someone else's cancer experience. This is not my intention at all. There is no good or easy cancer experience or treatment because there is no "good cancer," even though many of us diagnosed with breast cancer have been told exactly this. Breast cancer is the "good cancer." I don't think so. There is no hierarchy of cancer. It's all bad.

Cancer wreaks havoc on one's mind, body and spirit. The changes cancer brings may not all be permanent, but the physical and emotional scars can run very deep and may never entirely go away. They often remain etched into a person's psyche (and often the body too) for good.

Despite the horrors of all cancer treatments, there is something uniquely terrifying about the realization you need chemo. Just the thought of introducing toxic drugs into your body is unsettling. Knowing you are killing good cells as well as bad cells feels wrong and you can't help but wonder about the residual damage being done which may or may not be repairable. You can't help but wonder if you'll be paying the price someday down the road. Poison is poison. But of course, cancer doesn't let you look too far down the road. Cancer forces you to deal with the here and now. When chemo is your here and now, this can in some ways be more terrifying than hearing the words, *you have cancer.*

Information about the various chemotherapy drugs, side effects and managing such side effects is easy enough to find. However, information about how to mentally prepare and get past the fear before beginning chemo doesn't seem to be quite as plentiful. That's why I decided to write this book. I understand that fear. I felt that fear. Most importantly, I survived that fear. I want to help you do the same, survive the fear. I would like to offer my advice and suggestions for how you can enter into chemotherapy with a somewhat calmer state of mind and thus, hopefully help you to more easily come out on the other side in one piece, more or less anyway.

Can you actually mentally prepare for chemotherapy? Well, yes and no. You cannot truly prepare yourself for the unthinkable things in life, but you can understand a bit more about what to expect and this in itself is preparing. Obviously, I am no expert and I can only speak from my experience. This book is certainly not intended to be used as a replacement for any medical advice. I am merely sharing my experiences with the hope of helping you with yours. You have survived hearing the words, *you have cancer.* You will survive chemotherapy too.

Now let's start preparing.

2

GIVE YOURSELF PERMISSION

Even though I realized immediately after my bilateral mastectomy I would more than likely require chemotherapy due to unclear lymph nodes, I held out hope. Not until I heard the words from my oncologist's lips did I really believe it. Of course, that day came. I heard the words and that was a bad day. That was an ugly day. I was ugly, or rather my mood was, but now I realize that was okay and in fact, even necessary. That ugly day was a very important step in my processing. When you are forced to realize that you will be needing chemotherapy, it's okay to rant and rave a little, or a lot for that matter, and that's what I did.

I spent the entire rest of that ugly day vacillating between crying, thinking about crying, cursing under my breath and did I mention crying? I wanted to be left alone. I felt misunderstood and punished. Mostly, I felt sorry for myself. That was the day I did ask, *why me?* Here is an excerpt from my upcoming memoir which is taken directly from my journal entry written on the day I was informed chemotherapy was recommended to be part of my treatment plan. The fear and ugliness of my mood at the time is apparent and this is precisely why I chose to share it here with you.

I am unable to keep my tears dammed up any longer and they uncontrollably flood out. I do not even try to stop them any longer. I head for the solitude of my bedroom walls, small comfortable white chair and view of the towering white pine trees outside the window. I sit and cry. I rock back and forth, sob louder and feel relieved to be able to stop pretending to be okay. I am not okay. I am miserable. I am afraid. I am angry. I feel cheated and unlucky. I am full of ugly feelings of disgust, despair, helplessness and self-pity. Yes, I feel sorry for myself and I don't care.

Chemo terrifies me. The thought of drugs with unimaginable side effects gushing through my veins makes me shudder. I don't want to feel nauseous, have diarrhea, get mouth sores or rashes, feel weak with no appetite, be tired all the time and lose my hair. Such thoughts and fears overtake my mind and I am sickened by them. I am powerless to stop my tears. David (my husband) finally stops coming to check on me. Even he wants to stay away. I don't blame him. My mood is ugly. I am ugly. I want to get away from me. I want to get away from cancer, but I cannot.

David did try more than a few times to say things like, *we'll get through this too*, but I didn't want to hear that, not that day. No, on that day I needed to feel ugly. I needed to feel sorry myself. I needed that day to process.

I remember later that evening my older sister who lives out of state called and listened to me rant. She simply *listened* and I cannot emphasize enough how valuable and helpful that was to me.

"I'm so upset," I told her. "I admit it; I am feeling sorry for myself. I'll deal with everything tomorrow, but not tonight. Tonight I just want to feel miserable. I need to feel miserable."

"Of course you do," was all she said to me. That's it. In those few words, she gave me permission to feel my true feelings and I will always be grateful to her for saying those four simple words, for allowing me to feel what I was really feeling.

If you will be having chemotherapy, I cannot emphasize enough how important it is to give yourself permission to acknowledge and express your true feelings. If your loved one is having chemo, I cannot emphasize enough how important it is to give them this gift as well.

Give yourself permission to feel however you need to feel.

3

ASK FOR HELP

Once you come to terms with the fact that you will be having chemotherapy, it's time to get busy. I say this tongue and cheek, but also seriously. Hopefully, you will have a little time to get some things done before you begin your regimen and one of these things should be putting together a support team made up of anyone who is willing and able to help out.

I remember when I went into labor with my first baby, my obstetrician said to me, "This is going to be the hardest thing you have ever done physically."

He was right. Labor was hard, but it was over in less than twenty-four hours and at the end of it there was this beautiful and brand new baby to love. In comparison, chemotherapy went on for months, with the reward at the end being my extended life. I can honestly say chemotherapy was by far the hardest thing I've ever had to do physically and emotionally.

In some ways it was harder to face than my bilateral mastectomy, harder than childbirth, harder than reconstruction. It was just really hard.

Before beginning chemo, it's important to recognize this fact and make plans to get help. It's perfectly fine to expect the best case scenario. You may very well be one of the lucky ones who will experience few or even no side effects at all, but it's vital to have a plan in place if this does not play out. If you have young children, this is even more essential for obvious reasons. Don't expect your partner, or anyone for that matter, to step up and fill in all the gaps, not if you want your relationship to survive anyway. If you are single, you are going to need to rely even more on family and friends.

This is the time to stop taking care of everyone else, at least temporarily. This is the time to ask for what you need and to be as specific as possible in what you ask for. This is the time to ask for help when you don't get those offers and to not feel guilty about doing so. This is the time to accept meals from friends, allow others to clean your house and send somebody else out to shop for groceries. This is the time to delegate chores and responsibilities to anyone willing to help out. This is the time to call on family and friends. They probably want to help out anyway. Getting through chemo is now your primary job.

It's time to focus on *you*. It's time to ask for help.

4

DO YOUR RESEARCH

Once you and your doctor have decided you will be undergoing chemotherapy, it's time to start doing your homework by doing some research and asking some, okay, many questions. Actually, how much research you choose to do and how many questions you choose to ask is up to you. Some people want to learn as much as possible about their particular drug cocktail(s) and all the possible side effects and some are probably satisfied with knowing much less. Do what feels right for you.

My cocktail for the first couple of months was Adriamycin, the "Red Devil," along with Cytoxan. For the second half of my treatment I received Taxol. I wanted to know as much as I could about these drugs before they started flowing through my veins. Knowing gave me a sense of control at a time when I felt I had control over very little.

Generally, an oncologist will give you a handout outlining the particular side effects associated with your particular drugs. This will probably be pretty general as oncologists don't want to go into too much detail. If you're like me, you'll be busy Googling away on your own when you get home. Just be wary and be sure you stick to reputable sites that offer legitimate and reliable information. I like Mayo Clinic's site as a starting point. There are many others. When researching, take notes and make lists of questions to take with you to your next appointment. At this point your mind is too full to remember much, or at least mine was.

Be sure to spend adequate time with your oncologist getting all your questions, concerns and fears addressed. Again, take notes. If you have a partner, his/her questions are important too. You might need a separate list. Don't hold back. Ask anything, even if it seems trivial or embarrassing. This might seem obvious, but it's hard to feel bold and confident when you are feeling so vulnerable (health-wise) at the same time. It is the oncologist's job to explain things to you to your satisfaction. Think of him/her as working for you. If you don't understand something, ask for it to be explained to you over and over again until you do understand or feel satisfied. Try not to feel intimidated. Your oncologist has probably heard it all before and he/she cannot read your mind.

Also, don't be afraid to shed some tears while in the presence of your oncologist. This can be an emotional time. For some reason it was hard for me to allow myself to cry in front of my oncologist, or any doctor really. I always tried to hold myself together until I got home or was at least out of the clinic and in my car. There was one time when I was not successful at holding back the flood gates and I think my doctor was a little uncomfortable with my tears. In hindsight, who cares? That uncomfortableness was his problem. Your oncologist may need the reminder that cancer and chemo are both things we might need to cry about. Oncologists deal with this stuff every day. We don't, or haven't. Remember you don't have to be super-human, always putting up a brave front, not even in front of your oncologist, perhaps especially not then.

Finally, remember you have the right to know as much as you want to know about the mystery drugs that will be infused, injected or ingested into your body. You have the right to know what to expect.

Questions for Your Oncologist

- If chemo is not in a pill form, will I be getting a portacath (a small medical appliance that is surgically placed beneath the skin through which drugs can more easily be injected and blood samples more easily drawn) or will I be receiving chemo through an IV via a vein in my arm or elsewhere? Generally, a portacath is easier for the patient causing less discomfort than a needle poke each time. If you have a preference, opinion or choice in this, be sure to speak up.

- What drug(s) did you choose for my treatment and why did you choose them?
- How effective is this treatment?
- Do I have other options?
- What if I choose not to do chemo?
- Am I a candidate for a test such as the Oncotype DX test? (A test for some who qualify which gives a recurrence score and can help in determining if chemo should be part of your treatment)
- How will my sexuality be affected?
- If applicable, how will my fertility be affected and are there things I can do now to help me plan for children at some point?
- Will I be able to keep working?
- Are there prescriptions I should fill before my first chemo session?
- Who should I call (day or night) with questions that might arise?

Do your research and ask questions until you are satisfied with the answers.

5

CONSIDER TAKING A CHEMO CLASS

Unfortunately, by the time I needed chemo I was already far too familiar with the whole process. My mother had had chemo a few years earlier, though in hindsight, I now think in her case it was a mistake. As a result of her experience, I already knew quite a bit about the typical infusion and the typical side effects, if there is such a thing as typical, which of course, there is not. Despite my knowledge, when a class was offered to me and my family to inform and educate us about what to expect during chemo, my husband and I signed up. We figured, why not? We decided to offer the opportunity to attend the class to our college-age sons *if they wanted to attend.* They chose not to and that was fine with us. Some facilities have special classes for kids of different ages. These may or may not suit your family's needs.

Our chemo class was taught by one of the chemo nurses. We received a packet of general information, listened to a short lecture, watched a video, took a tour of the chemo room and had an opportunity to ask questions. Our chemo nurse instructor was quite knowledgeable, but somewhat lacking in the tact department, though I admit to being quite sensitive emotionally at the time. During the question and answer segment and in front of the whole class, she asked me what drugs I would be given and when I told her, she looked me squarely in the eyes and said, "Nancy, there's just no doubt about it. You will lose all your hair."

I found that remark to be insensitive and unnecessary. It seemed almost as if she was "rubbing it in" somehow, which of course she wasn't, but that's how it felt. On the whole, the class was worthwhile, the most beneficial part being the tour which did help to alleviate some of my fear about the dreaded chemo room. This was also another important opportunity to ask questions and get answers from a different source. After all, the chemo nurses have an entirely different vantage point than the oncologists and they can be an invaluable source of support and information. Take advantage of their expertise.

Now days many hospitals have cancer guides on staff who are trained in helping patients manage their cancer care. Such guides can also assist you in finding available resources that may help you with any aspect of your cancer experience. If you'd like such a guide, ask for one.

This also might be a good time to check out any available support groups. Some hospitals have groups for family members too. Many people find support groups to be amazingly helpful while others do not. You might find the camaraderie to be just what you need to feel less alone. Talking things over in a safe environment with others who have been there can be a life-saver. And don't underestimate the benefit of online support groups as well. No matter how you do it, connecting with others who understand during this time of great stress is vital to your well-being.

Remember this is the time to gather all the information you can, so consider signing up for a chemo education class if one is available. Make use of other available resources as well.

6

NOW ABOUT THE HAIR

If you are going to be receiving the type of chemo that does not generally result in hair loss, this can be a good thing as well as a bad thing. How can not losing your hair ever possibly be a bad thing you might ask? Well, when some people find out you are having chemo, but you are not or will not be losing your hair, they may be dismayed and for some odd reason less sympathetic. Somehow almost everyone equates chemo with hair loss. Many times this is the case, but not always. If you don't lose your hair, be prepared for insensitive reactions and remarks which can be frustrating to say the least.

If you are told you probably will be losing your hair, it's going to feel like a real punch to your gut. I don't know why we let our hair, or lack of hair, be such a big deal in this society, but we do and it is. Much of a woman's self-image and sexuality, no matter what her age, is very much related to her hair. This is just a fact. When you're a woman and losing your hair, it can feel like you are losing part of your femininity and this is really a hard thing to grapple with. Suddenly you feel literally, as well as figuratively exposed. People will say things like, it's only hair or it'll grow back in no time. This might be true, but saying these things is not helpful and, in fact, is hurtful as it minimizes the loss. Losing your hair is a loss. We grieve for things we lose, including lost breasts and lost hair. You are entitled to this grief.

If you are going to lose your hair, you will probably be inundated with stories about head-shaving parties, beauticians who make house calls to shave heads, letting the kids help shave it off and so on. While any of these strategies might be perfect for someone else, this doesn't mean they are right for you. I was not one tiny bit interested in throwing a head-shaving party. I did not want to make losing my hair into a fun and festive event. Nothing about it felt fun or festive and I wasn't about to pretend otherwise, but that was me. You might love those ideas.

The important thing to remember is taking charge, as far as you are concerned, does not necessarily equate with shaving your hair all off before or when it starts to fall out. You might feel more in charge leaving it alone and waiting to see what happens. That's what I did. I think I was rebelling against that chemo class nurse a bit who told me in no uncertain terms I would lose all of my hair. Well, in actuality I didn't, not all of it. I kept a fair amount at the nape of my neck, which was nice when I wore a baseball cap. I did maintain some nice "fringe hair" back there. Not shaving all my hair off when it started falling out made me feel more in control. I decided to wait and shave it off at the end of chemo. That's how I chose to "do the hair."

Of course, your decision might depend upon your job situation. No one wants to have clumps of hair falling out unexpectedly at a board meeting or over lunch. But no matter what, don't feel pressured about when to shave your hair off. In fact, it's not written in stone anywhere that you have to shave it off at all. You can certainly just let it happen as it happens. This just might be the best approach for you. Who knows? Only you do, that's who.

It's also worth mentioning that if you do lose the hair on your head, you will probably also lose the rest of your body hair. Your eyelashes, pubic hair, under-arm hair, leg hair and perhaps eyebrows will probably also disappear. No one really told me this part and in some ways, losing my eyelashes was harder for me than losing the hair on my head. Bare eyes are so, well, bare. The eyebrows often hang on more stub-bornly for some reason unknown to me, though they usually do thin out a bit, or a lot. You never know for sure what will happen.

On a slightly humorous note, during chemo and for a while after, I could never figure out why my nose was so runny. Then one day it dawned on me that all those little nose hairs were also gone, hence my runny nose. Never thought much about those little guys before. We take so many things for granted, even little nose hairs! Extra tissues might be needed.

Remember your cancer experience is yours and yours alone. Only you should decide what to do (or not to do) about your hair.

7

DO YOU WANT TO BUY A WIG?

Don't wait, shop early on

While I do not believe it's necessary to shave your hair off early on, wig shopping is another matter. Once you know your hair will probably soon be a thing of the past, if you choose to buy a wig, the sooner you do it the better.

First of all, the further you get into chemo, the less likely it is you will feel like going out to wig shop, or shop at all for that matter. As fatigue and other side effects kick in, you just might not feel up to the task.

The right color makes all the difference

If you want to shop for a wig style that is similar to your own hairstyle, obviously sooner is better than later. Another piece of advice is don't worry so much about matching up to your present style. The most important part of wig selection is choosing the right color. The right color can make or break how your wig looks, or rather how you look in the wig. I remember years ago when I was in high school, my mother purchased a couple of wigs (I'm not exactly sure why) and I always thought the colors were not right on her. They were way too dark. Unfortunately, I didn't have the heart to tell her and so I didn't. Her wigs would have looked so much more natural, and therefore better, had the colors been more appropriate for her complexion.

If possible, buy more than one

My next piece of advice is if you can afford it, buy more than one wig. It's nice to have two options. If possible, spend a little more on one and then buy another cheaper one for those whenever times. Some people prefer wigs made from real hair, but they are more expensive and I've been told more difficult to take care of as well. Just think of your own hair, is it really all that easy to take care of? Probably not. So the easiest and most economical way to go is the synthetic route. There are some amazing wigs available now. Take advantage.

Trying wigs on is a must

There are numerous catalogs offering very good

choices as well as some very good prices. If possible, I would suggest going to a store for at least one wig. Let's face it; everything looks great on a model in a catalog. You can't really tell how the wig is going to look on you until you try it on. I shopped at a Merle Norman Store and the experience was wonderful. Well, wonderful is a stretch. I mean I was shopping for a wig because I was going to have chemo and lose my hair, but you know what I mean. I tried on a lot of wigs in a lot of colors and the sales person was compassionate and extremely helpful. So much so I don't even mind "plugging" them here. Shopping at a retail store in person was the way to go for me. If you do decide to shop by catalog, be sure to check the return policy over carefully.

A second opinion comes in handy here too

Another suggestion is to take someone along with you when you shop for a wig. This might be your spouse or partner, a good friend, a sister, daughter or whoever. I took my husband because I knew he'd be brutally honest if need be and he was. Also, I figured he was going to be the poor soul looking at me the most, so he deserved a say in the matter. Try to find someone who will actually be helpful. You don't want someone who will just nod in agreement with you. This is one time when you need another voiced opinion, so maybe one of your more outspoken friends is the one you might want to take with you. Honesty is always the best policy and in this case, too, it's the only one worth having.

What about all those accessories?

When you buy your wig, it's also a good idea to buy one of those little head caps that fit under it. Strangely enough, I found they did help keep me cooler and minimized itching. Also, be sure to pick up some wig shampoo, a wig hairbrush and a stand on which to dry your wig after you wash it. As for other head gear, I did buy some bandanas and caps. I never could get the hang of scarves, but they look fabulous if you can figure them out. Caps are great, except for that little hole in the back that seems to scream "bald." Those fake bang fringes are not really worthwhile. Another thing to consider is getting something to wear at night. You will be surprised at how much chillier you feel in general with no hair on your head and unless you sleep with the covers pulled up over your head, you may very well feel cold at night. Plus, if you get up at night to use the bathroom, it can be quite startling to face your bald self in the mirror. Purchasing a nice, soft, cottony sleep cap easily and comfortably takes care of both issues.

Covering the cost

If money is tight, and it may well be, your cancer center should be able to direct you to an American

Cancer Society contact person who can direct you to someplace to go to get a wig for free. Some hospitals also have donation centers, so check out what they have. If you have some friends who want to help, this is a good opportunity for them. Ask them to donate some dollars to help you buy a wig. They might just jump at the chance to do something meaningful. And remember if you do have insurance, it might cover the cost of a wig, at least up to a set amount. Ask. If it does not cover the expense, be sure to complain and complain loudly. Remember if your insurance does cover the cost of a wig, you will need a doctor's prescription for one. A wig is generally referred to as a *cranial prosthetic*, a label that frankly, I found condescending and somehow silly and over the top, but...

How long will you need a wig? (If you choose to wear one)

Finally, I must admit I didn't wear my wigs all that much, but when I wanted to they sure were nice to have. I had a wedding the summer I was bald and a couple of other events to attend. It was just easier for me to go with a wig on. Also, remember you will still be bald for a while after chemo ends and it might be some time before you have hair you feel comfortable with. Some people don't give a hoot about going out in public bald or with only some peach fuzz up there, but if you do, wigs come in handy.

Ultimately, wigs are uncomfortable, hot and itchy; they are wigs after all. If you are able to buy one that fits right, you might be able to stand wearing it for a few hours at a time for those occasions when and if *you* feel the need.

Remember you do not have to ever buy or wear a wig just to please someone else. It's entirely up to you.

8

TAKE CARE OF YOURSELF

Hopefully you are one of those people who has been taking at least reasonably good care of yourself. If so, congratulations! Being more fit and strong as you begin chemo will only be an asset. If you're not one of those people, don't beat yourself up. Guilt is almost always a waste of time and energy. Get started now taking better care of yourself and do the best you can.

As I said before, chemotherapy will be one of the hardest things your mind and body will ever have to deal with. This is why it's so important to talk about the importance of proper nutrition, rest and exercise before, during and after chemo. Many others have addressed these topics, so I don't feel a need to re-hash what you probably already know about proper diet and exercise, however, the following points are worth stating and worth thinking about as you pre-pare for chemotherapy and try to get yourself into the best possible frame of mind.

Nutrition

- First of all, accept your body right now as it is. After all, you are fighting for its survival. How can you do this, if you don't accept it? I know, you feel like it's let you down a bit right now, but it's still your best friend and ally. Where would you be without it?

- This means don't worry about your weight right now. Your focus needs to be on eating as healthy as possible, period. Generally it's advised to try to keep your weight fluctuations to 5% or less in either direction, but don't obsess about your weight. Now is not the time.

- Do not choose this time to make radical changes in your diet. Your body will be going through enough trauma. Of course, it's imperative that you do attempt to make healthy food choices and unless you've been living under a rock, you know what these are. Your body will be depending on you to feed it the proper nutrients for rebuilding healthy cells, repairing tissues, fighting off infections and recovering from and coping with side effects.

- If you haven't been, start right now trying to take in enough fluids. Taking in enough fluids is always essential; during chemo it is even more critical that you do.

- Recognize the chemo process is cyclic and you may feel like eating less during the chemo phase (the first few days following treatment) and more during the rebuilding phase (the rest of the time until your next treatment).

- Consult with a nutritionist or ask your oncologist if you are unsure and want help with dietary needs. Use the resources available to you. *Again, ask questions until you are satisfied with the answers.*

Fatigue

The fatigue factor is a major side effect for many undergoing chemo. It's important to realize how hard your body will be working and you will need to rest or sleep whenever your body tells you it needs to, even if it's an hour after you just got up! There were times when I literally could not keep my eyes open even though it was mid-day or earlier. Of course there were also times when I couldn't seem to catch a wink of sleep despite feeling exhausted, another common side effect of anti-nausea drugs.

The fatigue factor is also why it's crucial to have help lined up, especially if you are parenting young children, trying to hold down a job, or both. Plan now. You might need to cut down your hours at work, so now is the time to talk with your employer.

Again, don't wait. Employers don't like surprises, so try to keep yours informed as much as you can while at the same time maintaining your privacy.

Exercise

If you have been exercising regularly before your diagnosis, again, congratulations! You are indeed a person to admire. You will probably be able to keep exercising, although perhaps not to the same level of exertion. If you have been more of an "onner/offer" like me, well, that's okay. Do plan on trying to fit some exercise in there somewhere during your day, even if it's only a walk to your mailbox or around your house. Studies are showing that exercise during chemo is beneficial in so many ways. No surprise there. The fresh air alone can work wonders.

On a side note, when I was going through chemo, I was going through reconstruction as well. It was also summer and often hot. Taking a walk sounded so easy, but it wasn't. Actually, the walking part was the easy part. It was the getting ready part that proved most challenging for me on many occasions.

I can't tell you how much I dilly-dallied around trying to figure out what to wear merely to walk down my own street. Like anyone would care what I was wearing, right? Admittedly, I was more than a little self-conscious about heading out the door after my bilateral. Tight or even semi-fitted t-shirts were out of the question, as were bras for a long time. I bought some button-down blouses, but so often those felt like something my mother or grandmother would have worn. Believe me, it wasn't easy to come up with something to wear, but when I did, I always felt better after my walk outside in the fresh air. The point here is, if you need to go out and buy something new to help yourself feel comfortable and more confident while exercising during chemo, well then do it. You deserve to splurge a bit.

Take care of yourself. Most importantly, be kind to yourself.

9

CONSIDER KEEPING A JOURNAL

I've always enjoyed writing. Since my cancer diagnosis, writing has become an even more integral part of who I am. I see writing as something to do for pure enjoyment. I also adamantly believe writing is a very therapeutic tool you can utilize to help yourself heal and grow. Writing may not heal your body, but it sure can help heal your mind. I believe writing, more specifically journaling, can help you get through chemotherapy. I believe journaling can help you get through anything.

If you have kept a journal or diary during anytime of your life, you've got a real head start at making your way through this maze that is cancer. If you have never journaled before, please keep reading and then at least consider giving it a try.

Why is journaling helpful?

Journaling forces one to think more clearly, or at least to think. Journaling revitalizes and almost always makes a person feel better. Journaling is visual proof you have accomplished something, felt something, survived something and maybe even grown from something. Journaling gives you confidence and inspiration to keep on going. Journaling is a personal record of a piece of your life and this cancer piece is like no other and indeed warrants keeping a journal.

When you are going through cancer, or any trying time in your life, journaling is a very powerful tool to help you cope, which unfortunately not enough people tap into. Journaling can help get you through the rough patches. Just seeing your thoughts and feelings written down somehow validates them, even if you are the only one seeing them. If ever there was a time when you needed your feelings validated, this is it. In a journal, you don't have to pretend to be positive, strong, brave or tough. In a journal you can feel free to tell your truth, all of it. There is something very freeing, empowering and healing about not holding back your true thoughts and feelings, even the negative ones; perhaps especially those. One could say that journaling is like having your own therapist literally at your fingertips, well almost!

Tips for getting started on journaling

- First decide what format you want to use. I still prefer to purchase my journals in book form because I like an actual visual "container" for my thoughts. Plus, a journal in book or notebook form has a more intimate feel to it later on and it's easier to not misplace, a problem I tend to have. If you prefer, you can certainly use your computer or other device.

- Try to set aside a few minutes each day or at least a few times each week to journal, so you get into the habit of journaling. It doesn't have to be the same time of day.

- Decide if your journal will be for your eyes only, or if others will eventually be allowed to read it. Personally, I don't think there's much point in writing a journal worrying about what others might think if they read it, but that's me.

- It might sound obvious, but do date each entry. Our memories fade fast and we won't remember them down the road. Plus, chemobrain is very real.

- If you have trouble getting started, simply record the date, weather, time of your doctor or chemo appointments, family events, how you are feeling or whatever. Everything in your cancer journal doesn't have to be about cancer.

- Think of journaling as an exercise for your mind, part of your treatment plan. You aren't wasting time!

- Tell yourself you are creating a written record about pieces of your personal cancer experience. You might not want to remember it now, but later on you probably will.

- Try playing relaxing music or lighting a candle while you journal.

- Don't judge what you write, just write...

- Make up prompts for yourself. For example, visualize yourself in retirement, on vacation, finished with chemo, or living the life of your dreams. Then just write...

- Be honest about your hopes, fears, dreams, frustrations and well, everything. Otherwise, what's the point?

After journaling for a period of time, go back and reread your entries. You just might be astonished by your very own words. You might be surprised how well and how much you have survived. This alone is very empowering.

I'm grateful for the safe sanctuary journaling provided me during my chemotherapy. I'm not sure how I could have coped without journaling. Journaling was how I coped. That's a powerful statement. My hope is that journaling will help you cope better with your cancer and chemo experience too. I'm confident it will.

So, what are you waiting for? Go ahead and get started on that journal. I promise you won't be sorry you did!

Consider journaling as a tool to help you cope with chemotherapy. Consider journaling to help you cope with your cancer experience period.

10

PLAN A GETAWAY, NO PLAN TWO!

Before you begin chemotherapy if at all possible, consider taking some time to just get away. Of course, you won't be able to completely get away; your mind won't allow this to happen, but if it's at all feasible, do try to escape somewhere for a day or two with a loved one or even by yourself. You don't have to take much time or spend many dollars. It's not even essential to leave town, just a change of scenery will do. Getting away briefly can help you "get your mind in order" and do wonders for your emotional well-being.

The weekend before I started chemo, my husband and I jumped in the car and took a leisurely three-hour drive to one of our favorite destinations, the North Shore of Lake Superior. There is something about Lake Superior that has a special calming effect on my soul. Maybe it's the name itself, Superior. It sounds exactly that, superior. The expansive body of water seemed to hold even more significant meaning for both of us at that time. The grandeur and beauty of Lake Superior quickly reminded me of my place in the greater scheme of things. That simple affirmation was somehow very comforting.

During that time away, we spent precious moments sitting on our private balcony marveling in the vastness and beauty of the ever-changing water, reveling in leisurely eaten meals in the restaurant, enjoying each other's company and just being a normal couple. It was as if we were in disguise and on a secret undercover mission of sorts. Time was standing still for us, if only for a couple of days.

One afternoon there was even a brief lovely wedding ceremony that took place directly below our balcony. The bride and groom and all their guests never once looked up, so they never realized they had two more unannounced wedding guests. Observing an intimate occasion, even as unnoticed and uninvited guests, was a nice reminder of the fact that life was carrying on. Normalcy was, well, normal.

There was a wonderful calming effect to that weekend experience and when we left at the end of it, both of us were indeed in a better place mentally to face whatever was ahead.

In addition to planning a mini-getaway before commencing chemo, I would also highly recommend planning something fun to look forward to when chemo ends. Again, it's really not the destination or the length of the getaway that matters. It's the act of separating oneself from the present illness/chemo situation that does. There is something very healing and conclusive about getting away again when chemo ends. Doing something concrete marks your survival of something very difficult and gives you an opportunity to tell yourself you made it.

If you cannot manage time away for whatever reason, imagine it in your mind. This works too and you get to imagine yourself anywhere. How great is that?

Getaways can serve as focal points or diversions when you need something pleasant to remember or think about during chemo treatment.

If possible, plan for some time away before chemo begins and again for when it's over.

11

DON'T FORGET YOUR PARTNER'S NEEDS

This chapter is one I hesitated to include in my book, but in the end I decided it was a topic that did merit a few words of discussion. It sounds like stating the obvious, but a cancer diagnosis has a profound impact on you as an individual, as well as a profound impact on your relationship with your partner. Any kind of stress impacts a relationship and the stress of a serious illness puts enormous strain on even the healthiest one. If you are in a committed relationship, in a sense you are both diagnosed. If you have a partner, in a sense you will both be going through chemotherapy and in a sense, you will both be experiencing the side effects.

After a diagnosis, some relationships will falter and even completely crumble. Some will hang on and survive, but barely. Still others will strengthen and grow into something even better. Then of course, there will be every possible variance in between. Perhaps some may not agree with me, but I don't think you can or should ignore your partner's needs during cancer treatment, including during chemotherapy. If you are the cancer patient, you definitely deserve to have the focus be on your needs; in fact, the focus must be on your needs. This doesn't mean, however, you can simply ignore the needs of your partner and I'm not just talking about sex. Intimacy and sex are important components to your relationship of course, but there is so much more to tend to.

Your partner still needs to feel cared for too. If you say hurtful things because you're frightened or angry during chemo, your partner still deserves an apology. If you are moody and irritable due to steroids or insomnia, your partner still deserves respect and consideration (and perhaps more apologies). If your partner is going above and beyond taking care of things, your partner still deserves a thank you. You need reassurance, but so does your partner. You're afraid. So is your partner. You still want to be considered desirable, so does your partner.

During chemotherapy, you and your partner will both probably still want intimacy of some kind and you will need to figure out what works for both of you. This might be a good time to discover some new means of pleasure giving. For example, consider giving greater emphasis to cuddling together or giving one another massages.

During chemotherapy, or anytime, the most important thing of all to remember is to communicate openly and honestly with each other. Do not pick this time to close down or withdraw, even though you might feel like doing just that. Do not pick this time to over-protect or shut out your partner, even though you might feel like doing both of these as well. Your partner cannot read your mind and you cannot read his/hers. Talking can work wonders and keep ill feelings from festering.

Also, *don't be afraid to bring the topic of intimacy and sex up with your doctors.* You can bet they won't bring it up if you don't. If they cannot help you directly, hopefully they can steer you toward someone who can.

Never settle. Relationships take work before cancer. Relationships take work during your cancer treatment. Relationships take work when cancer treatment ends.

Take care of relationships that matter to you.

12

WHEN CHEMO DAY ARRIVES

When the day arrives marking the beginning of your chemo campaign, expect to feel many emotions, the greatest one more than likely being fear mixed with plenty of dread. I remember that day well. I was terrified, but at the same time surprisingly outwardly quite calm.

I also remember the chemo nurse asked me before getting started, "Well, how do you feel, Nancy? Are you nervous?"

It wasn't possible for her, or anyone, to completely understand how fearful I was actually feeling. If truth be told, I felt like leaping out of the brown vinyl recliner I had carefully chosen and running out the door as fast as possible.

Again, this was why I wanted to write this book, to help alleviate some of your fear. If you know what to expect, at least somewhat, hopefully some of the fear can be tamped down a bit. Sometimes getting rid of even a little bit of fear makes a difference.

Before you begin chemo, your doctor may or may not recommend a port. If you have a choice in the matter, in my opinion, a port is the way to go once you get over the shock of needing such a God–awful thing. Generally, a port is surgically inserted on a day before chemo starts. It's a fairly minor procedure, but many like to get it out of the way early. My surgeon wanted to put my port in place a week or more before chemo started, but I bawled like a baby when he told me this because my husband and I had our getaway planned and the thought of going on our mini-vacation with a port in, caused me considerable distress. Go figure. I guess this was one of my breaking points. My tears and pleading quickly changed the surgeon's mind and my port was surgically put in place on the same day as my first chemo infusion. That worked out fine for me. Who said tears can't get you what you want? Just kidding.

You might find it helpful to have your partner, another loved one or a friend accompany you, especially for your first chemo infusion. Others prefer to go it alone. Decide before the day arrives. Certain drugs may make you too sleepy to drive safely, so find out beforehand if you'll even be allowed to drive home. It's usually a good idea to eat something before your infusion if you can, although they usually have soup, crackers, juice and the like available, so don't worry if you can't eat beforehand. Don't expect to sleep much the night before. Also, chemo takes several hours, so be sure to wear comfortable clothing.

When you arrive at the clinic or hospital for your first chemo infusion, generally speaking, here is what you can expect:

- You will check in with the receptionist like usual at your cancer center.
- Your weight will be recorded, as it will be closely monitored for fluctuations throughout chemotherapy.
- You will have an appointment with your oncologist either before or after your infusion to go over things and to have a quick physical exam.
- You will have blood taken to check and subsequently monitor your red and white blood cells, as well as other markers. If you have a port, blood can be drawn through that. I always liked to receive a copy of my blood work report. If you want one, ask for it.
- You will meet the chemo nurse who will be responsible for your infusion. He or she will double check your name and birthdate and help you get comfortable.
- Some cancer centers allow you to choose between a private room or a group setting. In a group setting, depending upon how busy your

facility is, there may be just a couple of others receiving chemo or a dozen or more. If you're put in a large group setting, there may be little privacy. This can vary quite a lot. Think about which you might prefer if you do get a choice. Be sure to ask about available options.

- You may very likely receive anti-nausea or pre-chemotherapy drugs first through an IV, again via your port if you have one. This usually takes about half an hour. In addition, you may also be given fluids to help drugs work more effectively and to keep you hydrated. Don't be afraid to drink fluids as well. Don't worry about bathroom breaks. You can easily use the restroom during infusions. Dragging the IV along with you is no big deal. Just be sure to ask the nurse the first time what you can and cannot disconnect.

- The infusion of your prescribed chemotherapy drug(s) will then begin. The process may take several hours to complete, so be sure to bring reading material or music to listen to. Some people sleep or watch TV. I could never do either.

- When the infusion is complete, your IV will be removed and your vitals may be checked again.

- Your oncology nurse should go over any possible side effects to expect and give you a chance to ask questions. If you have any, be sure to ask.

- You may receive prescriptions for anti-nausea drugs to take at home for a day or two. It's even better if you get these filled before your first chemo day. Be sure to fill all prescriptions and start taking medication(s) as directed before you feel ill. You want to stay ahead of the game and prevent side effects from developing if at all possible.

You're done! Next time should be a little easier. Now go home and try to get some rest, chemo is exhausting both physically and mentally.

Knowing what to expect on chemo day can help you feel more relaxed. Find out what you can expect.

13

AFTER YOU'VE BEGUN

Once you have formally begun your chemotherapy campaign, you will learn pretty quickly how your body responds. After a cycle or two, you will be able to predict at least to some extent what side effects seem to crop up for you. This is another helpful benefit of journaling. You will figure out which days you feel more like eating and which days you just want to sleep. You will begin to figure out your digestive patterns and if there are certain foods you want to avoid. You will learn how your bowel habits are affected. You will probably even figure out when you are most likely to feel moody or edgy. As you begin to figure things out and as some of the mystery of chemo starts to wane, or rather when you start realizing you can handle the mystery, it becomes at least somewhat less frightening, but it will always be unsettling.

There are plenty of good resources and helpful (as

well as non-helpful) information abounds on the internet about chemo, side effects, managing them and so on. I chose not to cover these things in this particular guide. However, one of the best resources I found and would like to share about is a book called, *The Chemotherapy Survival Guide: Everything You Need to Know to Get Through Treatment, Third Edition*, by Judith McKay, RN, OCN and Tamera Schacher, RN, OCN, MSN. I found it to be concise, accurate, practical and user-friendly. It helped me tremendously and was an easy-to-go-to reference when I needed to look something up quickly.

When you are going through chemotherapy, people (even loved ones) will say things to you that will be downright irritating. You will miss out on some things you generally enjoy. You will have down days. You will feel like crap at times. You will not get everything done you want to, not even close. You will feel guilty at times for taking your loved ones along with you on this "ride" no one wanted to be on. You will feel angry and sorry for yourself from time to time. You may, in fact, experience a whole range of unexpected and unfamiliar emotions that you aren't supposed to be feeling. You may feel as if the end of chemotherapy will never come and be highly irritated when others tell you you're almost there or that you "only" have four treatments left. You may very well feel like you can't make it through the day much less the next four treatments. You may feel nothing at all like the brave warrior society seems to want to portray you as. You may be totally unsure of how you do feel. *During chemo, uncertainty and emotional upheaval thrive.*

I'm here to tell you such feelings are normal. *You* are normal. Never let others tell you how you should be feeling during *your* cancer/chemo treatment. Don't try to fake positivity or pretend to feel what you do not. Be true to yourself and allow yourself to feel whatever it is you are feeling. This doesn't mean get stuck or wallow in self-pity. No, but do acknowledge your feelings and then decide how to move forward or sideways (and occasionally backward). If you need professional help to sort things out, get some. Above all, speak *your* truth. Share *your* truth. When others don't understand, help them to understand by communicating honestly with them. Chances are they will understand, or try to. Give them the opportunity to do so.

I'd also like to reassure you that you will still have good times even during the depths of chemo. You will have good days, hopefully lots of them. You might have few side effects or even none at all. You will still be able to do things you enjoy. You will still be able to go to parties and attend functions if you choose to do so. I remember going to a movie during my chemo regimen and laughing out loud during the middle of it. The sound of my own laughter startled me as I realized, yes, I *was* having a good time. I could still laugh at a silly movie and forget about things for at least a couple of hours. That simple realization felt really good.

During chemotherapy (and after) it's really important to surround yourself with people who love and accept you. Do things that bring you joy. Take a drive. Get lost in a good book. Listen to your favorite music. Walk the dog. Try a new hobby. Reach out to an old (or new) friend. Learn something new. Attend a support group meeting. Plant or buy some flowers. Be extra kind to yourself. Heck, start writing a blog - I started www.nancyspoint.com during my chemo. In a word, live! That's the whole point isn't it?

Finally, it's important to remember that once your initial cancer treatment ends, you will be entering another new transitional phase in your cancer experience. You will be turned loose and more or less expected to figure out your "new normal" (another phrase I don't much care for). For some, this phase proves to be the most challenging one of all. You may very well feel as if you've been thrown into yet another "sea of uncertainty," because in fact, you have been. But that's another book…

During chemo (and after) be gentle with yourself and do things that bring you joy.

AFTERWORD

I hope this guide has been helpful to you as you face the prospect of chemotherapy for the first time. I also hope you are feeling slightly less fearful after reading it and have learned a thing or two. A cancer diagnosis is a lot to deal with. Cancer treatment of any kind is a lot to deal with. Chemotherapy is a lot to deal with and then some. Hang in there. You'll make it through this too.

Of course, there are no guarantees in life, or in cancer treatment. We all hope we will not require further treatment. We also all know some of us will. Finishing chemotherapy, or any other kind of cancer treatment, does not mean you are cured for good. It does not mean you might not require treatment again someday. However, finishing this particular round in the ring is no small accomplishment.

Once you are diagnosed with cancer it's never over, but you have made it this far. You'll make it through chemotherapy too.

Finally, thank you for reading my book. Good luck with chemotherapy and beyond!

What lies before us and what lies behind us are tiny matters compared to what lies within us.

ANONYMOUS

ABOUT THE AUTHOR

Nancy Stordahl is a free-lance writer and former educator. She resides in Wisconsin with her husband, two dogs and one cat. She has a daughter and two sons. After her breast cancer diagnosis in 2010, she began writing a blog at www.nancyspoint.com where she candidly discusses her own breast cancer diagnosis and treatment, reconstruction, hereditary cancer, grief/loss and the under-discussed challenges of survivorship. She also shares her concerns about some of the forms of breast cancer awareness and advocacy and is a staunch advocate for those living with metastatic disease. Nancy has had articles accepted for publication in numerous venues, is a featured blogger for Huffington Post and continues to work on her upcoming memoir.

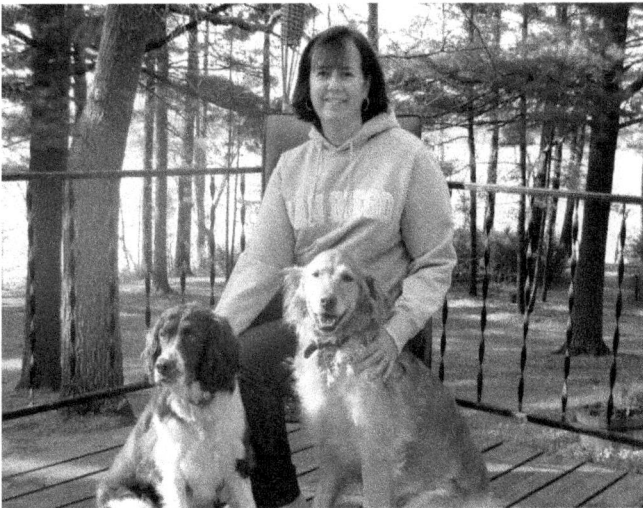

NOTES AND QUESTIONS

NOTES AND QUESTIONS

NOTES AND QUESTIONS

To read more or to contact Nancy Stordahl
please visit
www.nancyspoint.com